Why growing numbers of parents are choosing
natural *immunity for their children*

by Forrest Maready

Besides historical references, the names, places, and accounts mentioned in this book are used anonymously. Any resemblance to actual persons, living or dead, is entirely coincidental.

Text copyright ©2018 by Forrest Maready
Cover typography ©2018 by Forrest Maready

FEELS
LIKE
FIRE!

All rights reserved. Published in the United States by Feels Like Fire, an imprint of Feels Like Fire.

ISBN 978-1722908690
Printed in the United States of America

Also by Forrest Maready:

The Autism Vaccine, 2019
The Moth in the Iron Lung: A Biography of Polio, 2018
Crooked:Man-made Disease Explained, 2018
My Incredible Opinion Vol. 1, 2016
My Incredible Opinion Vol. 2, 2017
Massa Damnata, 2017

unvaccinated

Why growing numbers of parents are choosing
natural *immunity for their children*

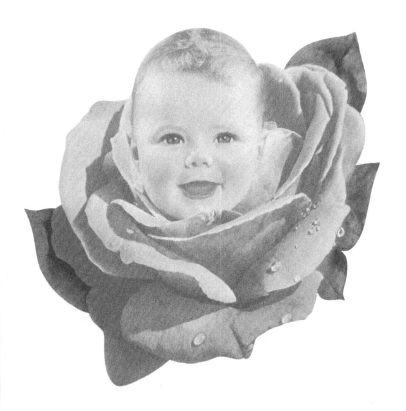

Forrest Maready

Unvaccinated?

"You're going to do what?" I asked a friend as I picked up my jaw from the floor.

He had just told me that he and his wife were going to skip all vaccines for their child, and I couldn't believe it.

"All of them?" I asked again.

"All of them," he said, confidently.

I couldn't wrap my head around it. He never talked about 9/11 conspiracies or government cover-ups. He was a smart guy—in fact, he had just completed medical school, and somehow had come to the conclusion that he and his wife were not going to allow any vaccines for the precious baby growing in her womb.

"What an idiot," I thought to myself. "Why would you take such unnecessary risks with your baby?"

Anti-vaxxers were crazy people who believed in UFOs and somehow ignored all scientific evidence that suggested vaccines were the greatest medical invention humanity had ever created—responsible for the conquest of most diseases and millions of lives saved. Why would anyone with half a brain purposefully avoid this miracle medical intervention?

In the weeks and months that followed, I began to look more closely at the debate. I had heard of Andrew Wakefield and a debunked scientific paper that linked autism and vaccines. I knew that actor Jenny McCarthy had received a lot of flak for speaking out about autism and vaccines. Beyond that, I knew very little. My son had received vaccines as a child—many more than I felt comfortable with. Personally, I had always avoided the flu shot, as I had seen many of my friends come down with the flu whenever they got one. Did that make me an anti-vaxxer?

I remembered poking fun at one or two friends who expressed concern about vaccines. I equated their reluctance to a fear of needles, or the stress from having to physically restrain their child. As I began to read more, I realized how little I actually knew about the topic. My mind swirled with confusion as some of the stories I had absorbed over the years appeared to be different than what I had been taught.

It was an incredibly uncomfortable experience. When something you *know* to be true, without a shadow of a doubt, begins to take on a much different shape in your mind—it's not something most humans are well-equipped to handle. As a few things I *knew* to be true about vaccines appeared to be much less clear, my world was shaken.

"How could this be?" I asked myself. "If this is actually true, then how could I not know? How could doctors not know this?"

I read the endnotes and looked up the references. I looked up the references of the references. I continued down the rabbit-hole for months until I realized that much of what I had heard about vaccines and disease was mostly wrong. Again, this was a deeply troubling journey and the only reason I believe I was able to sustain it was because I had a natural curiosity much stronger than my fear of the unknown.

It is now years later, and I have dedicated my life to trying to help people understand the truth about vaccines and disease. I have made over 130 videos, written four books, and traveled across the country. I have sabotaged my professional career and made enemies of many of my family and friends in the process. All in an attempt to help people understand the true pros and cons of vaccines.

I didn't start speaking about vaccines for fame or fortune, because there is none. I simply wanted others to see what I had realized—without having to invest the years of research and mental anguish. This short book you are now reading is just a quick "dip in the pool" on the subject. It is my sincere hope that everyone who reads this will begin to research the truth about vaccines and disease—and in the process, create a huge improvement in your family's long-term health.

Just as importantly, I hope that any fear and anxiety you may be feeling about this subject will disappear after reading this book. Vaccines are a contentious topic, and it can be intimidating to believe something many of your friends and family disagree with you on. Just know that the people I've met who've taken the plunge and are not vaccinating their children are some of the healthiest, happiest, friendliest people I know.

I'm so glad you've decided to challenge yourself by

pulling back the veil and looking at something from a slightly different angle. I don't expect this book will completely change your mind about vaccines, and that's not the point. As long as you are able to search for the truth and make an informed decision based on those facts, I'm guessing you and your family will have an incredibly healthy future.

What is an anti-vaxxer?

What does "anti-vaxxer" even mean? Is it a negative term meant to humiliate someone, or is it just an informative label meant to describe someone's beliefs? Anti-vaxxer can mean both of those things—and everything in between. Many people are opposed to all vaccines, no matter the situation, while others have skipped or delayed particular vaccines for certain children. You may have already delayed a well-child visit because your child was sick. Everyone is different and has a different situation.

The first "truth" you should become comfortable with: Many people who are called anti-vaxxers are not anti-vaccine at all, but simply voice their concerns about vaccines. Some feel like there are too many, while others may choose to follow a more lenient vaccine schedule from another country, such as the Netherlands. Still others may skip booster shots for a previous vaccine because their child developed a problem.

Here is a good way to think of people like me:

Anti-vaxxers want fewer vaccines — as few as possible.

Other people have no problem with the 72 vaccines children are suggested to receive in the United States, and would have no problem if many more were added. Anti-vaxxers are the opposite. We are constantly trying to figure out how to provide a healthy upbringing for our children with the fewest vaccines possible. Zero would be ideal.

I will talk more about ingredients later, but just understand that I think of vaccines like chemotherapy. You would probably never give your child chemotherapy *before* they had cancer, even if you were told it might protect them if they happened to get it later on in their life. Why? The chance of them getting cancer is so low, you'd probably rather not expose them to the trauma of chemo in the off-chance they might need protection in the future.

You may think this is a poor analogy because chemo is much worse than vaccines. I thought that too, at first. I thought vaccines were harmless shots—

like Tylenol in a syringe. We will find out the truth is much different. The ill effects of chemo stop soon after you stop taking them. Because vaccines are designed to alter your immune system *forever*, the side effects of something going wrong can also last for a very long time.

As a result, anti-vaxxers take the risk/benefit analysis of vaccines very seriously. Here are the main factors that might go into an anti-vaxxer's decision to delay or skip a certain vaccine:

- The chance of contracting the disease.
- The chance of permanent harm from the disease.
- The likelihood a vaccine will actually work.
- The chance of permanent harm from the vaccine.

There are very few people who *randomly* decide to forego vaccinations for themselves or children. Unless they were raised in a family that did not vaccinate, most people spend hours researching the risk versus the benefit of certain vaccines and diseases before they make a decision to skip a single one. Unfortunately, there are others who had something bad happen to their child after being vaccinated. Many of these people didn't need any research to be convinced of their danger.

After considering these factors, there are growing numbers of people who have decided to delay, skip or avoid certain vaccines altogether. Some of them are refusing all vaccines—even the big ones like polio. If you are shaking your head in confusion and anger right now, that's okay! Hang on to that thought for just a few minutes—the stories we have been told growing up make it seem idiotic to skip these vaccines. Once you start looking a little deeper into the actual facts, the truth is a bit different than you were likely told.

The one chart

As I began to study vaccines, the single biggest surprise came in the form of a chart in a book called *Dissolving Illusions*. I'll never forget the confusion this chart created in my head. All my life I'd heard vaccines saved humanity from horrible things like smallpox and polio. Before vaccines, there was widespread death and destruction from disease. After the vaccines, all of the childhood illnesses that had plagued humanity for centuries disappeared— basically overnight.

This is the chart that changed everything for me:

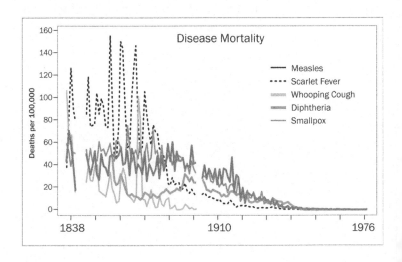

It showed how many people were dying from a couple of different diseases over the last 150 years. I couldn't believe what it suggested: every disease was getting less deadly at the *same* time. The thing that blew my mind was that one of the diseases didn't even have a vaccine. But it didn't matter—the mortality from all of them was going down in sync. I thought that either the data contained in this chart was fabricated, or the stories that I'd been told were wrong. The chart starts back at 1838, so there are some data gaps in places, but in general, the mortality from the 5 diseases on this chart were trending downwards well before vaccines were invented. I thought the author must have been using some statistical trick to look at deaths in a weird way that would get the result they wanted, but after a lot of investigation, I realized it charted deaths per 100,000 using government data sources.

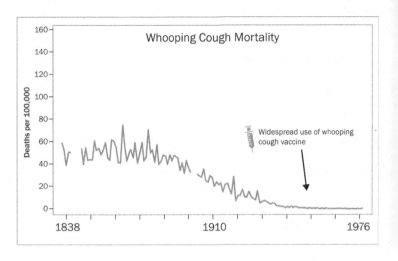

What was really shocking for me was Pertussis—also called Whooping Cough. The mortality from this disease was basically zero *before* the vaccine was even invented.

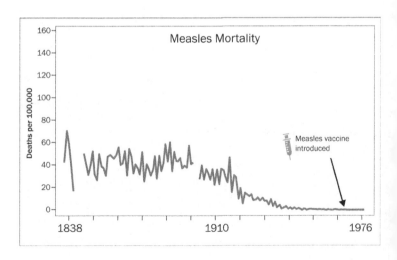

Measles was the same way. These are two diseases that we still vaccinate for today and the mortality from them had fallen to nothing *before* the vaccine. Then the book pointed out the 5th disease on the graph—Scarlet Fever:

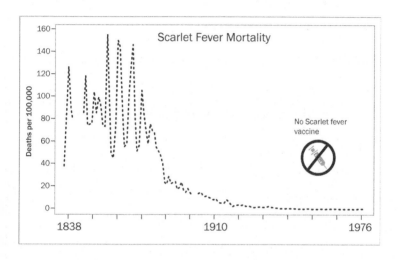

Scarlet fever is different than the others because they never developed a vaccine for that one. Like the other diseases, it became less and less deadly over the past 150 years—even though it didn't have a vaccine at all. All of these diseases—plus many other ones without vaccines—followed a similar decline.

I had grown up believing the smallpox vaccine eradicated smallpox, and that the polio vaccine saved kids from being paralyzed, so I assumed these other diseases would have a similar trajectory—horrible deaths *before* the vaccine was invented, *then* a decline in death. How was it these diseases had become so trivial before—or without—a vaccine?

As it turned out, people began to understand how disease was spread. If someone caught an infection, authorities could contain it by isolating that person and keeping them away from others. This meant disease outbreaks became far smaller. There were also improvements in food safety, hygiene, and sanitation that meant all of the health woes typical of life in the 1800s disappeared.

The biggest reason was the most shocking to me. All throughout the 1800s and into the 1900s, medical care was so horrible it often killed far more people than it saved. People began to realize that arsenic and mercury were probably not the best medical treatments to be giving infants and sick people. This move away from metals as a medicinal treatment helped save many sick people. Through improvements in living conditions and medical care, many of the diseases that were "killing" thousands of people eventually became trivial infections that no one feared, *before* most vaccines were even invented.

At that point, I felt like maybe I needed to rethink some things. I had heard stories of parents saying their kids developed autism soon after their vaccines, and I knew there were some rare side effects here and there. But if the diseases weren't really killing anyone, how bad were the vaccine's side effects? How often did they happen? Was SIDS really just a baby that died randomly with no explanation at all? Were food allergies really from ingredients in the vaccines like some people suggested? Everywhere I looked, the story was not the one I had been told as a kid, as an adult, or as a new parent.

Take a look at the chart and decide for yourself—either the chart is a lie, or maybe all of the improvements in medical care, sanitation and nutrition—maybe *they* had more of an impact on human health than anything else. If that is true, it ought to make you begin to question many other things you thought were true about vaccines.

Measles

After I spent days researching the data sources for those graphs, manually typing in the numbers from the reports into my own Excel spreadsheets to see if they matched, I finally gave up. I had to accept something that, for me, was very difficult: many of the diseases we now vaccinate for ceased to be deadly long before vaccines were ever invented for them. Other diseases—for which vaccines were *never* developed—followed the same trajectory.

It was so confusing. I had been told that vaccines saved us from all of these diseases, but the cold, hard data showed they had very little to do with the huge decline in deaths from disease. If you're like I was, you're probably shaking your head right now, trying to figure out where the disconnect is. Someone must be lying about something, right?

Think about measles for a minute. If you're younger, the only thing you may have heard about measles are stories on TV about scary outbreaks. Just a few decades ago, measles was considered a trivial illness—

just like a cold any kid might catch during the winter. It was a rite of passage for every child and was routinely joked about on TV shows like the Brady Bunch. However, once a vaccine was developed for the disease, health officials and doctors begin to speak of the infection as a terrifying event—mainly because most people weren't scared enough of measles to get the vaccine.

What do anti-vaxxers think about measles and the vaccine? The measles vaccine *does* work for some people. It *does* create some protection from a measles infection. You may feel like this is an unexpected statement coming from an anti-vaxxer, but let me reiterate an earlier point I made: our goal is as few vaccines as possible. To do this, we need to accurately calculate the risk versus benefit from every vaccine to maximize the chance of having a healthy child. Many of us don't have a fanatic devotion to avoiding vaccines—we are simply calculating risk and benefit in hopes of having the highest chance of good health. Just like you, we have no desire to put our children needlessly at risk.

There are vaccines that *do* work—with a very large

asterisk. They are a hack, an attempt to cheat mother nature at one of her best tricks—immunity from future attacks of a particular bacteria or virus. You see, vaccines *can* create a type of immune response, but it's often much different from catching the disease naturally. As a result, vaccines don't work exactly the way we'd like. They also don't protect for very long. A natural infection typically gives you immunity for life, whereas a vaccine only works for a few years— sometimes not at all.

Certain vaccines *will* have an impact on measurements of the disease. For measles, the vaccine *did* affect the number of children coming into the doctor's office with a measles infection. It *did not* affect the deadliness of the disease. Apparently, certain people with pre-existing health problems unrelated to measles are likely to have trouble with a measles infection—whether they are vaccinated for it or not. These people may really struggle with what would be a harmless infection in other people.

This is why measles is still a problem in third world countries. It is *not* because they have a shortage of measles vaccines, but because these countries have many people who are severely lacking Vitamin A. In developed countries, this deficiency isn't a problem and you almost never see anyone dying from measles —not because they're not catching it, but because it's just not a deadly disease in healthy people.

The measles vaccine didn't move the needle on measles deaths in the U.S. If you vaccinate your child for measles, they will require frequent boosters for the rest of their life to be considered truly protected. Because anti-vaxxers are trying to minimize the number of vaccines their children receive, many opt out of the measles vaccine. The disease is, for most, a trivial infection, and in its natural state will create immunity for life—no boosters will ever be needed again.

If you're following along, you may agree with me, if only partially. You may be thinking, "Sure, some of the more obscure diseases stopped being deadly before the vaccines came around, but what about polio? You cannot say that the polio vaccine did nothing to save children from death and paralysis."

Polio was a big stumbling block for me. I had gone through the chart and finally came to the conclusion that perhaps vaccines didn't play as big of a part in the prevention of disease as I had thought. But polio, I knew—there was a disease in need of a vaccine if there ever was one. How could anyone in their right mind not get their child vaccinated for polio? The answer to that question blew my mind.

What about Polio?

Polio is probably the most famous disease we vaccinate for. Everyone can recall images of children in braces and people lying inside iron lungs before the vaccine. Anyone who grew up in the 1940s and 1950s probably knows someone in their family or neighborhood that was affected by this horrible disease.

As the story goes, in the 1950s a vaccine came along, and the disease disappeared. You stopped seeing children in braces, and the iron lungs became a thing of the past. A heroic story of man over microbe that no one can deny, right? I became so obsessed with this story, I ended up writing an entire book about it, *The Moth in the Iron Lung*. The truth about polio, is not quite as simple as we were told and is decidedly more horrible than you can imagine.

Polio is a nickname for *poliomyelitis*, which means inflammation of the grey matter of the spinal cord. If you get a lesion on your spinal cord, that part of your body may develop paralysis. This disease nearly always occurred in children, which is why it was called *infantile paralysis* for decades. It almost always started in their legs, and as lesions continued to move up the spinal cord, they would lose control of their abdomen, their arms, and finally the muscles that expanded and contracted their lungs.

If they could not breathe, they would die. The iron lung, first introduced in the late 1920s, helped children who were paralyzed in such a way to breathe. This was a godsend because some children could eventually recover from their paralysis—as long as they could keep breathing. The iron lung bought many of them enough time to survive until the lesions went away. They might have residual paralysis and difficulty walking, but they would live, and for many, have completely productive lives.

Polio was basically non-existent before the 1800s. There might have been a case here and there, but you really don't see it in the medical literature until the 1890s, when it began to appear in *epidemic* form. Some people will point to an Egyptian painting of a man with a cane and a shortened leg as evidence that polio always existed, but as we will soon see, there is no way of knowing what caused this man's condition.

As it turns out, the paralysis of poliomyelitis can be caused by many different things. Several viruses can cause it, as can several different bacterial infections. Surprisingly, pesticides could also cause it. Studies were conducted in the late 1800s with a popular pesticide called Paris green. They purposefully fed animals too much pesticide and it paralyzed them in their "hind quarters"—just like what was happening with children. Scientists did autopsies on the animals, found lesions in their spinal cords, and pronounced they had died from poliomyelitis, or polio—from pesticide poisoning.

The pesticide contained a metal called arsenic, and may explain why many parents originally referred to polio as *teething paralysis*. A popular medical treatment at the time was "teething powders," a concoction given to infants who were teething. They contained massive amounts of a similar metal— mercury. Teething powders became popular in the early 1800s and appeared about the same time you start seeing isolated cases of polio. Coincidence? You decide.

It became clear that certain viruses and bacteria could also cause paralysis, but only if they got inside the nervous system. For all of human history, these microbes had never caused problems, but starting in the late 1800s, they suddenly gained the ability to get into the nervous system.

This likely had something to do with a new pesticide that was invented in 1892—lead arsenate. It was a combination of lead and arsenic and was sprinkled and sprayed on many fruits and vegetables that were later eaten. It's popularity was due to the fact it couldn't easily be washed off with water—an advantage for farmers who didn't have to re-spray after a storm, but a decided disadvantage to mothers trying to clean their children's food.

It appears that not only did this metallic pesticide create paralysis through direct poisoning, but caused a leaky gut issue in children that allowed different viruses and bacteria to pass through the intestines and into the spinal cord directly behind. Remember that humans had lived with these viruses and bacterial infections for hundreds of years with no paralysis until the late 1800s. Within a year or two of the invention of this new pesticide, polio began to appear in that same area of the country.

In the 1940s, at the end of World War Two, a new pesticide called DDT began being used by nearly everyone and polio became much worse. Unlike lead arsenate, which was sprayed on food, DDT was sprayed directly onto children in an attempt to protect them from flies and mosquitoes. Ironically, it was thought these insects could transmit polio, and DDT was sprayed on children *to prevent* polio. Many people from this era will recall chasing the DDT truck down the street, frolicking in the clouds of pesticide trailing behind—another popular pastime that no doubt contributed to the paralysis of that era.

By 1952, people began to stop using DDT because many insects had already started to develop resistance to it. Parents also began to suspect it was more toxic than they had been told. At the same time, cases of infantile paralysis, or polio, began to plummet. 1952 was the peak for polio cases in the United States—not just the kind caused by the poliovirus, but the paralysis due to *all* of the other viruses, bacteria and direct pesticide poisoning. They *all* began to disappear as DDT stopped being sprayed on nearly everything.

Even though all types of infantile paralysis began to go away after 1952, most history books will say it's because of the Salk polio vaccine. This is just not true. The vaccine worked very poorly, and most of the public didn't even get it until years later. It was officially introduced in 1955 but was quickly withdrawn because it was inadvertently causing paralysis due to manufacturing problems. Many didn't get a polio vaccine until years later, when a different, presumably safer version of the polio vaccine, the Sabin oral polio vaccine, came out in 1961.

By then, polio had all but disappeared from the United States. As it turns out, even the new vaccine wasn't actually needed. Polio had nearly vanished by then. It had appeared suddenly in the 1890s alongside the introduction of the pesticide, lead arsenate, and had suddenly disappeared in the early 1950s alongside the abandonment of DDT. The story we grew up hearing left out many important parts. The paralysis of polio wasn't just caused by one virus, but many different things—all of them tied directly to the wreckless spraying of pesticides that began and ended in lockstep with the appearance and disappearance of polio.

I realize this may be very difficult for you to digest, but just to demonstrate the reality of what happened, I want to tell you about a scientific study that was conducted in Detroit in 1960. Because the initial polio vaccine worked so poorly, scientists were concerned. In an attempt to understand what was wrong, they took stool samples from almost 1,000 people who had been diagnosed with polio that summer. They did thorough testing on all the samples and determined that less than one third of the people that had been diagnosed with polio actually had polio. They had been paralyzed by one of the other viruses, bacteria or acute pesticide poisoning.

This was the main reason the first polio vaccine wasn't working—the people didn't even have polio at all! They had been paralyzed by one of the many other causes of paralysis that appeared in the late 1890s and disappeared in the 1950s. It didn't matter that many of them had received 4 or more injections of the polio vaccine—they weren't paralyzed by polio, but something else.

If you have trouble believing this story, I'd recommend you look up "The Present State of Polio Vaccines," a paper that covers the conference in 1960 where scientists and vaccine manufacturers were attempting to understand what was happening. It is an eye-opening account of the confusion happening behind the scenes of the polio vaccine.

Today, countries that still use dangerous pesticides like DDT continue to struggle with infantile paralysis, also known as polio. They have controlled some of it with the polio vaccine, but remember, the vaccine only addresses a single cause of paralysis—the poliovirus. Because there are many other microbes capable of paralyzing, other forms of infantile paralysis have increased nearly just as much as poliovirus-caused paralysis has decreased. If they were to clean up their environment and stop using these dangerous pesticides, all forms of infantile paralysis would likely disappear just like they have in other countries.

This is why anti-vaxxers skip the polio vaccine without the least amount of concern. We know that there were many different causes of the paralysis of polio and that without massive amounts of ingested pesticides, no one is likely to have a problem. Even if we lived in a country where DDT or lead arsenate ingestion *was* a problem, we realize that the polio vaccine only protects from the poliovirus infection, and none of the several other viruses or bacteria that could also cause paralysis if given the same opportunity.

The narrow focus of the polio vaccine on the poliovirus, when many other microbes can also cause paralysis, actually represents a much bigger problem with vaccines—one that actually gives many anti-vaxxers comfort in skipping other shots for their children.

Too many shots?

Recall that most anti-vaxxers prefer as few vaccines as possible for their children—zero if possible. There are some vaccine manufacturers that would of course prefer you take as many as possible. I would assume most people, and this may include you, want a commonsense number of vaccines—no more or less than what is reasonable.

How do we decide what is reasonable? The obvious path would be to decide what diseases are problematic, and if there is a vaccine for them, make a decision as to whether the risks and cost of administering the vaccine outweighs the risks and cost from the disease. Sounds fairly simple, doesn't it?

The vaccines most children receive today are not decided on in this way. Many shots on the schedule are diseases which were once problematic many years ago, but due to improvements in sanitation and medicine ceased to be a problem—*before* vaccines were developed for them. They were added simply because a vaccine had been successfully produced. It's like the old saying, "When you have a hammer, everything is a nail."

Some vaccines are physically combined with other shots simply because the manufacturer can get away with it. It is certainly more convenient to get one injection instead of three, but when the other two are not vaccines you really need, it feels like you are being taken advantage of. Because vaccines contain some ingredients we'd rather not inject in our children unless absolutely necessary, these combo vaccines pose a big problem.

Depending on how you count, the current childhood vaccine schedule in the United States suggests around 72 vaccines for your child. This is more than any other country in the world. Why is this? Does the U.S. struggle with more diseases than other countries? Is our sanitation and medical care inferior? Not at all. The government agency that creates the vaccine schedule knows that other countries are likely to follow their guidelines and as a result, works hard—alongside their pharmaceutical colleagues—to add as many vaccines as possible to the schedule.

For example, most countries don't recommend the Hepatitis B shot administered to infants at birth in the United States. The vaccine was originally developed for drug users and other people at a high risk for Hepatitis B. Because a pregnant woman is routinely tested for this disease, her newborn (who is not likely to be sharing intravenous needles) can confidently be ruled out for this shot. But in the U.S., every infant born in a hospital is routinely given this vaccine, minutes after birth, even if the mother tested negative for the disease.

This vaccine wasn't put on the childhood schedule because Hepatitis B was killing thousands of infants in the United States. It was put on the schedule because there weren't enough high-risk people opting for the shot. Even if the Hepatitis B vaccine was an innocuous shot with little risk, I would find it objectionable. Stabbing an hour-old infant in the foot or leg and injecting something into them for no reason bothers me. Unfortunately, the Hepatitis B vaccine contains aluminum—an ingredient that we will find out is something you would never want injected into your child.

So far, few other countries have followed this outlandish practice. If you have a baby in nearly any other country, they would not dream of injecting a one-hour-old infant with a Hepatitis B vaccine. The mother would have been tested for it, and as the disease is nearly always the result of sharing drug paraphernalia or unprotected sex, the infant is unlikely to get it. In the U.S., if you choose to do what most other countries do and avoid this vaccine for your child, you will be called an anti-vaxxer.

The chickenpox vaccine is another example of a vaccine that exists on the childhood schedule solely because of overzealous government health officials and industry lobbyists. Chickenpox is a trivial childhood disease that parents had no fear of. In fact, many children were purposefully sent to neighborhood "parties" with other infected children in hopes of their children catching chickenpox. No one—besides perhaps the pharmaceutical executive— was begging for a chickenpox vaccine. After it was created, it was predictably added to the recommended childhood schedule.

Like Hepatitis B, many countries don't recommend

the chickenpox vaccine. They gladly allow their children to get chickenpox naturally and enjoy a lifetime of immunity—for free and with essentially no risk. In the United States, if you choose to do what most other countries recommend and skip this shot for your child, you will be labeled an anti-vaxxer. Are you beginning to see why I embrace the label?

Making informed decisions about your child's health can be challenging. There are many shots on the childhood schedule that are trivial diseases no one wanted a vaccine for in the first place. Others are holdovers from fifty years ago that haven't been removed simply because they make the manufacturer extra money and no one has complained loudly enough.

When you see many of these shots aren't necessary at all, and are simply padding the wallets of pharmaceutical companies, you may begin to question all of them. Take a page from many European countries: their children receive far fewer vaccines than U.S. children, yet they aren't suffering massive outbreaks of deadly disease. What do they know that we don't?

What disease do you fear?

Ask yourself something: What is the disease you fear most for your child? Without going on the internet and doing a search, what springs to mind? Think of the one disease you dread your child getting. Most people will say polio. Others may say whooping cough.

Think about this for a second—can you name a disease you are afraid of that doesn't have a vaccine? It's difficult for most. You may say Ebola or Zika, but most people can't name a disease they are afraid of that doesn't sit on the vaccine schedule. Why is this?

It is a strange phenomenon, but many people only fear the diseases listed on the childhood vaccine schedule. Do you fear tuberculosis? It's estimated to kill 1.7 million people each year. There is a vaccine for it. You could go get your child vaccinated for tuberculosis right now—a disease that kills millions of people each year—yet hardly anyone in the U.S. gets the vaccine *or* is afraid of tuberculosis. Why is that? It's not on the childhood vaccine schedule.

Think about measles. Measles was considered a trivial disease—even joked about on television shows. Decades later, now that a vaccine has been developed for it and is recommended for every child born in this country, public health officials and news media outlets lose their collective minds when someone comes down with a case of measles. Measles is *much* less dangerous than tuberculosis, but despite having vaccines for both of them, health officials and media reporters only seem to care about the one on the childhood schedule.

Chickenpox is the same way. A popular news show from the Netherlands recently featured a segment about picture day at the local kindergarten. This picture day was thought to be especially cute because nearly every child had chickenpox—their faces covered in dots. The photographer and teacher all came in to school, each child smiling for the camera, as if nothing was amiss.

Meanwhile, in the United States, where the vaccine is strongly suggested, news outlets cover a single chickenpox infection with the somber tone of a mass shooting. Children might be kept from school for weeks, despite the fact everyone is supposed to be protected from infection by the vaccine. In the Netherlands, the chickenpox shot is *not* recommended and they treat an outbreak as a humorous, even joyful, story. In the U.S., the vaccine is strongly recommended and stories of the corresponding disease outbreak are treated as ominous threats to public health.

I'm not suggesting there is some kind of secret conspiracy to make you fear the diseases we have vaccines for, but when you see the pattern over and over again, it does begin to make you wonder. Why should we fear diseases we have vaccines for— shouldn't it be the opposite? Shouldn't we fear the diseases we *don't* have vaccines for?

The unfortunate reality behind this phenomenon is most parents don't like vaccines. Most kids don't like vaccines. This is understandable. They are painful injections that often make your arm hurt and possibly feel sick. But there is an underlying fear that goes beyond temporary pain. For many parents, vaccines just feel wrong. There's something unnatural about restraining a screaming child against their will and allowing someone to inject foreign material into their body.

If parents didn't have a lot of fear regarding these diseases, many would just skip the shots. So public health officials and the media work overtime to create and maintain fear of the diseases we have vaccines for —just to make sure you don't skip any. You will notice, that besides Ebola and Zika, they rarely spend time reporting about diseases for which there are no vaccines (Ebola and Zika vaccines may be licensed any day now).

Some health officials will admit that a bit of fear-mongering is necessary because the vaccines made us forget how bad the diseases actually were. This is clearly not the case with the Hepatitis B or chickenpox shots, and many other diseases weren't feared before vaccines were invented for them. If anything, we fear these particular diseases *more* now than we did before their vaccines—largely due to the scary stories the media produce to foment fear. This fear begins to feel so strange when you see how other countries respond to outbreaks of some of these diseases—look up the Netherlands chickenpox outbreak when you have a moment. Watch how they laugh about it.

This may seem like a strange phenomenon unconnected to your opinions about vaccines, but for anti-vaxxers, it actually plays a very important role in our goal of giving as few vaccines as possible to our children. If you would have asked me years ago what the one disease I feared my child getting, it would have been polio. Once I realized the likelihood of my child getting paralyzed was nearly zero because we don't coat their food in DDT or lead arsenate pesticides anymore, I felt completely confident in skipping the polio vaccine.

If you took polio off the list, I'm not really sure what I would have mentioned next. Nothing would have come to my mind—I would had to have looked over the childhood vaccine schedule and picked something. You may be afraid of the diseases we have vaccines for, but here's a very important thing to remember: there are thousands and thousands of other viruses and bacteria which could harm your children just as easily. We have vaccines for just a tiny percentage of known viruses and bacteria—probably less than .01%, yet you could probably not name a single one. You are afraid of the ones listed on the childhood vaccine schedule, but not the others.

If a child were to be harmed by one of these other viruses or bacteria, it would be unlikely to make the news because there is no vaccine for it. If it were a "vaccine-preventable disease," then it would be talked about for days on end. Anti-vaxxers recognize this phenomenon, and realize that even if their child received every vaccine available on the planet (even more than the 72 recommended by U.S. health officials), it would still only protect them from a tiny fraction of the hundreds of thousands of varieties of microbes they might encounter any given day.

Instead of subjecting their children to potentially hundreds of injections, anti-vaxxers focus on creating optimum health and nutrition. We believe that vaccines can interfere with proper immune system function and know that when optimum health and nutrition are present, the immune system can take care of nearly any infection—even the ones for which vaccines don't exist.

At this point, you may be thinking, "Why can't I do

both? Why can't I give my children the vaccines that are available *and* focus on their health and nutrition for the other diseases which have no vaccine?" There is a specific reason for this, and I've held off talking about it so as not to scare you away. The reason most anti-vaxxers avoid a certain vaccine isn't only because they don't fear that disease, but two other reasons you'd probably never expect.

Unnatural

Although many of the vaccines on the childhood schedule could easily be considered unnecessary because the disease no longer poses a threat, many anti-vaxxers choose to skip some of them for another reason: *vaccines screw up your immune system.* This may come as a surprise to you, but our attempts to hijack the immune system with vaccines tend to create unintended consequences.

Most people think of vaccines as simply taking a harmful virus or bacteria, killing—or weakening it—so that it can't harm, and introducing it into the body to create an immune response without all the danger of getting the actual disease. Many vaccines don't actually work this way.

Take the pertussis, or whooping cough vaccine, for example. The pertussis vaccine—the "aP" in the DTaP vaccine—presents a really interesting example of how vaccines are inferior to natural infection. During a pertussis infection, the bacteria triggers the release of several toxins. One of them is extremely clever and is called ACT. ACT tricks your immune system into thinking nothing is wrong for about 14 days. This gives the infection a two-week head start before your immune system figures out what's really going on. During that time, the infection has time to get a solid foothold. Eventually your immune system catches on, and is able to develop protection against the ACT toxin. That's a good thing, because the *next* time you get a pertussis infection, your body will be prepared and the ACT sneak attack won't work. The *next* time you get an infection, it can be cleared easily because that two-week grace period will be gone.

When you receive a Pertussis vaccine, your body's immune system gets programmed incorrectly. The Pertussis vaccine doesn't contain any ACT—because they haven't figured out how to include that yet—so the vaccine forces your immune system to react to a pertussis infection differently than a natural infection. How? It reacts much more slowly.

Unfortunately, your body will never learn the 14-day ACT trick once you're vaccinated. Even if you get a pertussis infection after you were vaccinated for it, your immune system has already been programmed incorrectly from the vaccine and can't be taught the correct way—ever! It can't un-learn the old way. This is why it's so important to have the correct immune response the first time. You basically get one chance to get things right. I'm oversimplifying this a bit, but the crucial component of the natural immune response to whooping cough is your body's ability to quickly recognize that specific toxin, ACT, and start mounting a defense. The vaccine specifically prevents your body from doing this, ever.

Another interesting thing about ACT—you may have heard that many whooping cough outbreaks happening around the country actually might come from a *different* strain of bacteria than the one targeted in the vaccine—what they call *bordetella parapertussis*. This new strain may have been created from the vaccine itself, kind of like how antibiotics can create this same problem. The ACT trick is also used by the new strain of pertussis bacteria to get a two week head start on your immune system. If you had a natural pertussis infection, you will have developed ACT immunity correctly and would be able to fight off *both* infections, even though you were never vaccinated for bordetella parapertussis (because a vaccine doesn't exist for it). Nature is amazing like that.

Every vaccine is different, but nearly all of them have one or more problems like this. Nothing in life is free, and by trying to cheat mother nature's most complex invention—the immune system—we nearly always get something we didn't ask for. You may have seen recently how certain viruses like measles and polio are actually being used for cancer treatments? This just goes to show you how complex the interactions between the body and microbes can be.

Because we don't fully understand what kinds of problems vaccines may be creating with our immune system, and because these problems typically last *forever*, many parents are opting out of certain vaccines rather than risk permanently screwing up their children's ability to fight off infections (or possibly even cancer).

Finally, when you begin to understand how they work, you may come to this realization: vaccines are just gross. We have fewer McDonald's and more Panera Bread stores everywhere. We have Trader Joe's and Whole Foods everywhere. We have organic food restaurants and hybrid cars. All because people are more concerned than ever about what is going into their bodies.

If you were to take the ingredients in a vaccine and stick it on the label of a food product at Whole Foods, *no one* would ever buy it. It's not organic. It's unnatural. It is decidedly the opposite of everything that many of us fight for our children every day. The only reason people allow it is because they fear disease more than the vaccine itself. Hopefully, from what I've told you so far, you don't fear the diseases as much as you did.

While manipulating your children's immune system in ways we can't totally control may make you feel uneasy, there's one other very big reason many anti-vaxxers avoid certain vaccines. It's not just because they're unnecessary, and it's not only because they screw up their children's immune systems. It's because they contain ingredients the human body was never designed to deal with.

Ingredients

Many vaccines contain metals—on purpose, not by accident. Mercury has been a popular medicinal ingredient for two hundred years and was only recently recognized as being dangerous enough that it needed to be removed from vaccines. Mercury, or Thimerosal, is still sometimes used as a preservative in multi-dose vials of flu shots. Multi-dose vials are bigger and have a thin piece of rubber on the top called a diaphragm that keeps the vaccine inside free from contamination.

When a nurse or doctor draws up a vaccine by putting a syringe through the diaphragm in the vial multiple times, the chance of introducing something that shouldn't be in there increases. Thimerosal was added into these vaccines so if something got past the diaphragm, it would die—because mercury is toxic to all forms of life. Not a comforting thought for something you might inject into your child. Many vaccines used to come in multi-dose vials, because it was cheaper that way. Nowadays, most vaccines come in single-use containers. Because they will only be used once, you don't need the mercury anymore.

While Thimerosal has long been thought to cause neurological problems associated with vaccines, the danger of the aluminum they contain is only recently being understood. Aluminum is not a preservative—it serves a different purpose and is included in many vaccines regardless of whether they are in multi-dose vials or not. Aluminum has been in vaccines for a long time—since at least the 1930s—and its purpose is to aggravate your immune system into a stronger response. This is called an adjuvant.

When I say aluminum, you're probably thinking of aluminum cans being melted down into silver liquid and dripped into a vaccine. The aluminum used in vaccines is actually called a metal salt, and looks like a white, crystalline powder. It's still aluminum and is put in vaccines because your body hates it—your immune system reacts very strongly to it.

Because many of the components used in vaccines have been manipulated to the point they are less dangerous to inject, your body doesn't even see them as invaders and doesn't react to them. Aluminum is added because it forces your body to react to the vaccine. They don't *want* to put aluminum in there, but they *have* to. The vaccines will not work without it.

We've long known this ingredient to be dangerous. It's used in scientific experiments to help create *asthma* and *food allergies* in animals. It was shown as far back in 1921 to cause lesions in the cranial nerves —crucial components of your nervous system. The argument for their use has always been that vaccines contain such tiny amounts of aluminum that it couldn't be dangerous. People will tell you you eat more aluminum every day than what is contained in vaccines. This *is* what people thought twenty years ago, but recent scientific research has made it clear why tiny amounts of aluminum in vaccines can be so harmful.

For starters, toxins that you eat, or ingest, rarely make it past your intestines. Although humans ingest a small amount of aluminum in their diet, only about .3% of it is actually absorbed into the body. Ingested aluminum is in an *ionic* form that is easily filtered by the kidneys and can be stopped from causing neurological damage. The aluminum that's *injected* with vaccines is in a different form called *nanoparticulates*. This form of aluminum is much different than the ingested kind and creates a couple of problems you will never see with the dietary kind.

If you were to take the aluminum contained in a single pediatric vaccine and inject it into a specific part of a child's brain, possibly their *pineal gland* or the *area postrema*, they would almost certainly die. The amount of aluminum in many of the shots children regularly receive is toxic enough to kill anyone if it was administered directly into the wrong spot.

The safety with injected aluminum was always thought to be in its dilution. The dose might be deadly—we knew that—but it was assumed it was evenly distributed around the body rather than one specific place where it might cause serious problems. Think about pouring Kool-Aid powder into a pitcher of water. It spreads out on its own, and only needs a little bit of stirring to mix it evenly throughout the water. We thought the ingredients of vaccines would spread out evenly throughout the body in that same way. Unfortunately, it turns out we were wrong.

Until recently, we made the logical assumption that the less aluminum the vaccine contained, the less of it might make it into dangerous areas of your body. If the amount of aluminum contained in the vaccine was so little, then the chance of a significant portion of the metal reaching your brain would be infinitesimally small.

A terrifying discovery about aluminum was made recently: less aluminum is worse. Less aluminum is more dangerous. In the study, researchers injected mice with varying amounts of aluminum. Across the study, mice who received less aluminum per injection fared worse—their behaviors indicated neurological problems and the amount of aluminum that reached their brain was much higher. The mice that receive the two higher dosages of aluminum seemed to have less significant effects.

How could this be? When a vaccine is injected into your arm, the aluminum triggers an aggressive immune response and your body begins to mount an attack against it. This is often why your arm gets so sore after a vaccine—it's your body forming granulomas around the ingredients—a collection of fibrous tissue doing their best to wall off ingredients from the vaccine.

Scientists now understand that your body responds more aggressively with these granulomas at higher concentrations of aluminum. It makes sense when you think about it—the more dangerous the invader is perceived to be, the more aggressive the response. If you get a large dose of aluminum, the body works hard to wall it off inside protective granulomas. But the opposite scenario is more concerning—if the injection contains a smaller amount of aluminum, there is less granuloma formation and more of it makes it into your lymphatic system and blood. And if it gets into your lymphatic system and blood, it can get into your brain.

This was a stunning revelation that should have caused everyone to rethink what were safe amounts of aluminum in vaccines. Unfortunately, most health officials and physicians act completely unconcerned. Their websites have not been updated to reflect these new discoveries, and they'll shrug their shoulders if you mention it to them. If history has shown us anything, it is that those in authority will *always* be the very last to admit they were wrong. I wouldn't expect vaccines to be any different.

For most anti-vaxxers committed to as few shots as possible, most of us would never allow aluminum-containing vaccines to be administered to our children. The chances of neurological injury from the accumulation of aluminum from these shots is simply too high to be worth the risk from *any* disease. With aluminum being so strongly implicated in the brain damage of autism and Alzheimer's, I wouldn't recommend anyone—children *or* adults—take any aluminum-containing vaccines either.

Manufacturers know aluminum is dangerous. They've been searching for an alternative for decades. But metals aren't the only questionable ingredients in vaccines that should make you think twice about injecting them into your children. There are a few others. It's natural to ask, "Why do they allow these vaccines on the market? If they're truly that dangerous, why are they even allowed at all?" The answer to this question shocked me more than all of the others.

Safety

With any product, particularly medical products, there can be danger. Within a free and open society, there are two release valves which work in the consumer's interest to protect them from harm: safety-testing and lawsuits. Reasonable government regulations should require that the product be properly safety-tested before being released to the public. Secondly, if a product—despite passing rigorous safety-testing—is still causing harm, the company that manufactures that product can be sued for damages—an effect which should both compensate those harmed by the product, *and* force the manufacturer to fix the problem to avoid future lawsuits. Unfortunately, through purposeful manipulation of the system, neither of these release valves exist as they should with vaccines.

Let's take a quick look at the first issue—safety-testing. Vaccines are not classified as drugs, and as a result, can be safety-tested much differently than a typical pharmaceutical product. In a drug safety trial, a group of patients is given the true drug and another group are given a placebo—an inert substance that is incapable of causing a problem, such as saline. The trial might run for months, even years, to discover any negative effects the drug might be causing.

Because vaccines are not considered drugs, their safety trials are run much differently. Rather than looking for problems for months or years, they might look for a few days, and in some cases the trial may only last 48 hours. There is no rule for the minimum amount of time required to look for problems, so they will obviously run the trial for as short of a time as possible. It's infinitely cheaper that way, and problems are much less likely to appear.

If someone in a 48-hour vaccine safety trial began to notice a problem two or three days after they received the vaccine, this event will likely not be considered as caused by the vaccine. The effect of this tiny window of observation is obvious: for a vaccine to be blamed for any safety issue, it has to happen nearly instantaneously—an unlikely occurrence.

A second problem with vaccine safety trials—those conducting the trials claim they can't use a true placebo because it would be unethical. Why? They will say purposefully denying someone a vaccine to protect them from disease is not fair to that person. Despite the fact that the trials run for only days—after which the person would be free to get whatever vaccines they wanted—vaccine manufacturers claim that to deny someone *any* vaccine for those few days during the trial would be too risky for the patient. So rather than running a useful study by administering half of the group a saline placebo, they administer an existing, already licensed vaccine and compare the results of the new vaccine against that one (a vaccine which was also likely approved under a similarly flawed trial).

This is a practice so asinine you will probably assume that I am attempting to mislead you. You may be thinking, "Maybe this happened once or twice and you're making the suggestion that all trials are run this way." I will ask you to do a study on vaccine trials yourself. Don't trust what I'm saying. Look them up yourself and you will find they are nearly all run this way. One large trial testing the much-hated Gardasil vaccine *did* employ a tiny saline placebo group but relied on an aluminum-only injection for its main placebo.

The inevitable result of these two things is the illusion that every vaccine is safe. The test is unlikely to pick up adverse events due to its short duration, and even if it did, comparing it against another vaccine is likely to create a similar number of problems. If it *were* compared against a truly inert, saline placebo, the contrast would be much more pronounced.

There are other tricks the clinical trials employ to improve the appearance of safety. They kick out anyone who has any health condition at all. As a result, the health profile of the trial participants doesn't resemble the general population, but a super-human race of perfectly healthy creatures. If someone does develop an issue during the trial, doctors might be encouraged by those running the trial to diagnose the issue in such a way as to appear as if it were a pre-existing condition. If this happens, the participant is kicked out of the trial and their issue is never recorded as a negative event against the vaccine.

One of the most concerning things about these

safety trials is they are rarely conducted on babies or pregnant women—the two groups of people most often receiving vaccines and the most vulnerable to their ill effects. You can look through the 25 or so flu vaccines currently licensed in the United States and not a single one of them has ever been safety-tested on pregnant women, despite routinely being administered to them. The same holds true for the TDaP shot given to pregnant women. The fact that doctors inject pregnant women with this vaccine every day without a second thought gives me nightmares.

Finally, you should know that the vaccine schedule has never been safety-tested. Different vaccines have gone through these fraudulent safety trials as standalone products, but never together, as administered. Many babies will receive six, seven, sometimes eight or more vaccines in one visit. Combining so many injections like this without having tested them together would never be attempted with any other pharmaceutical product. The possible interactions between various drugs would be carefully studied and monitored. With vaccines, it's assumed there is no upper limit to the number an infant can receive simultaneously, and the possibility of cross-reactions between their various ingredients has never been studied.

Because of the way vaccine safety trials are conducted now, it wouldn't matter. Even if the full schedule were tested, it would be run as fraudulently as the stand-alone products currently are. It would not be tested against a true placebo, and the trial would run for mere days before being shut down and declared a success.

Again, you are probably having a difficult time believing this is true. I have done the research along with some of the best scientific minds in this field and can assure you, this is the reality of vaccine safety in the United States at this time. Great efforts have been made to raise awareness about this travesty, but the pharmaceutical industry is the most powerful lobby in government and is not going to allow proper vaccine safety to be conducted at this time.

I mentioned there were supposed to be two release valves designed to protect consumers from harm regarding potentially dangerous products. The safety trials regarding vaccines are a complete joke and should not be relied on for any meaningful data. What about the second release valve—lawsuits? If the way in which vaccine safety trials are manipulated doesn't make your blood boil, I can guarantee you the way in which vaccine lawsuits are conducted will.

Lawsuits

In the 1980s, an increasing number of SIDS (Sudden Infant Death Syndrome) deaths began to be associated with vaccines which had been administered just days, sometimes hours, earlier. While scientists and doctors have never officially declared a cause for babies that die suddenly without any apparent reason, many parents insist that immunizations triggered their baby's death.

The DTP vaccine, long considered to be one of the most dangerous shots, was often implicated. In 1979, four children from Tennessee had died within 24 hours of their first DPT shot. It turned out all of the children had received vaccines from the same production batch. Parents were fuming mad and the news media began to pick up on the stories.

Lawsuits began to pile up and vaccine manufacturers saw the writing on the wall—they would not be able to defend themselves from these lawsuits and be able to stay in business. They did something extraordinary that has never happened in any other industry or product—they threatened to cease manufacturing of vaccines if the government could not protect them from lawsuits.

Astonishingly, their demands were heard and met. In 1986, a piece of legislation, called the National Childhood Vaccine Injury Act, was signed into law to great fanfare by Ronald Reagan. With the introduction of this new law, vaccine manufacturers could no longer be sued for problems caused by their childhood vaccines. They were protected by the government. It called for the creation of a special court where vaccine injury cases would be heard— again, nothing like this exists in any other industry that I'm aware of.

If the court decides that a death or injury was due to a vaccine, the court will pay out a maximum of $250,000. This money does not come from the manufacturers themselves, but a special fee included in the cost of the shot—paid by *you* each time you or your child receives a vaccine.

Fast-forward 32 years later, and it's clear the court has become a nightmare for parents of children harmed by vaccines. Families are forced to suffer through sometimes years of litigation—all in hopes of getting a maximum of $250,000. Many of these cases never even make it to court because doctors are so insistent the recent appearance of a child's seizures or other problems had nothing to do with their vaccines.

The court is very selective in the scientific data it allows and, by all appearances, serves the role of protecting pharmaceutical interests from damage. Although settlements paid by the court are not coming out of the manufacturer's pockets directly, the court's unspoken job is to protect even the appearance of problems with vaccines. If they were to allow many of the plaintiff's cases to win, it would encourage other parents to file their claims. Even so, the court, which hardly anyone is even aware of—even by doctors and nurses—has paid out over $3.5 billion dollars since it began.

As a result of the 1986 National Childhood Vaccine Injury Act, vaccine manufacturers have been given blanket immunity from any problems their vaccines may cause. Only a fool would believe this would somehow *increase* the safety of the products they make. In reality, it has done the opposite.

Manufacturers have no incentive to properly safety-test their vaccines. They can't be sued if something goes wrong, and the safety trials are worse than useless.

Combined with stern recommendations from the government that every child receive the very vaccines manufacturers can't be sued for, it has created a unique and profitable situation for pharmaceutical companies. No other industry on the planet is afforded this protection—and for good reason. The ability for companies to be punished for creating dangerous products is one of the foundational mechanisms for keeping consumers safe from harm. Imagine the government requiring you to feed your baby a particular formula—breastmilk not allowed—while at the same time preventing you from suing the formula manufacturer for any problems their product caused in your baby. You might really start to wonder who was watching out for you and your child, wouldn't you?

With laughable vaccine safety trials and complete protection from lawsuits, I hope you will understand why anti-vaxxers are so reluctant to take vaccine manufacturers and their public health colleagues at their word. After having read about multiple cases of twins dying from SIDS the same night—sometimes the night after their well-child visit, I really began to question what might be causing these mysterious deaths. When so many parents have insisted their children came down with other strange problems just days after their vaccines, I started to listen.

Perhaps you're beginning to think vaccines may not be such a safe or necessary thing. Perhaps you're considering delaying or skipping some of the 72 vaccines the U.S. government insists your children receive. If you speak to anyone about this, they will likely mention another reason that you must vaccinate your children—herd immunity. You may be surprised to learn that the way herd immunity actually works is much different than what you've been told.

Herd Immunity

Herd immunity. It's a term that's thrown around like a weaponized guilt trip. They'll tell you, "Okay, you may have unvaccinated kids, but the only reason you're able to safely do that is because everyone else is vaccinating theirs."

Herd immunity is not what you've been told. I'm going to explain why, but just think about this for a minute: tetanus is not a contagious disease. You can't "spread" it, and you can never develop immunity to it. But the vaccine is required for many jobs, schools, or summer camps—supposedly because of herd immunity!

We've already seen how the threat of most infections had plummeted to nearly zero before many vaccines were invented. The paralysis of polio was related to massive pesticide poisoning and isn't a problem in countries that use safer pesticides. There are very few infections that pose a danger in a first-world country with modern healthcare. Anti-vaxxers avoid vaccinating their children not because they rely on others getting vaccines, but because they don't fear common childhood infections, they know how to treat it if their children did happen to get one, and they are thoroughly informed about the risks of side effects from vaccines.

Another common herd immunity plea: "You must get your child vaccinated to protect the weak and vulnerable from disease." This is a very powerful argument that attempts to appeal to your civic duty and the natural human compassion we all have. In reality, it doesn't play out the way most people think.

For starters, there are very few people who are truly "immune-compromised," meaning their immune systems are so weakened that they cannot receive vaccines. When I say very few, I mean almost none. Statistically speaking, you'd be lucky to encounter more than one in the course of a year of your life. If you were to encounter one of them, you would also have to simultaneously be infected. And not just infected, but infected at the stage where you are capable of transmitting the disease to other people (which is usually just a small window of time within the course of infection). If all of these things lined up, you might inadvertently get someone sick.

Unlikely to ever happen, but again, this call to protect the weak and vulnerable is constantly announced as a reason your healthy child should receive dozens of vaccines—not just to protect them, but the immune-compromised around them.

There's a big problem with this—some vaccines can inadvertently trigger the very disease they are designed to protect against. This is because some vaccines contain a modified version of the *live* virus. If you get vaccinated for a disease with a live virus, you are purposefully creating an infection. Ideally, it's a very mild form of the disease, but sometimes, things go wrong and the vaccine will cause a full-blown infection—a phenomenon called *shedding*. This is not a completely obscure event, and in fact, is the main source of polio in many countries today—from the vaccine itself!

You may already be aware of this concept but don't realize it. If you go to any children's cancer ward, you are likely to see a giant warning sign at the entrance warning anyone who has recently been vaccinated to stay away. They know that some vaccines can shed and create the very infection they were intended to protect against. So much for vaccines protecting the weak and vulnerable!

The final plea you hear about herd immunity involves the number of people that have to be vaccinated to keep deadly outbreaks of a disease from happening. For measles, they constantly say at least 95% of country needs to be vaccinated to keep this "horrible" disease at bay.

A few years ago, there was a measles outbreak that started in California's Disneyland. It was blamed on anti-vaxxers causing the number to drop below 95%. No one died, and of the 150 or so people that became infected, over half of them were fully vaccinated for measles—a curious fact that is not often mentioned in the news.

I want to explain why the herd immunity concept is completely ignored by anti-vaxxers. Herd immunity originally started as a concept to try to talk people into getting the measles vaccine. In the 1960s, they had just finished developing the vaccine, and because measles was considered such a trivial disease that no one was afraid of, no one wanted the vaccine.

Scientists did some math and said if just 55% of people were to get the measles vaccine, they could eradicate measles within two years. Vaccinate 55% of people, and the remaining 45% wouldn't even matter —the disease could be eradicated.

Remember, measles was a fairly trivial disease—no one feared it. There were very few deaths because of it, but it *was* a nuisance—missing school, etc. So they thought eradication would be possible if they could hit the herd immunity number. After a few years of hard work, they were able to hit their vaccination target of 55%, but measles didn't go away like they thought it would. People were still getting infected. So they upped the number to around 70%. Eventually, they were able to hit 70% of people vaccinated, and *that* didn't seem to do the trick either. Since then, health authorities have continued raising the herd immunity number to 80%, then 85%, then 90%, then 95%—where we're at today.

Between 90 and 95% of the US has been vaccinated for measles for a long time, yet we still see measles outbreaks. What's going on? Why isn't herd immunity working like we thought?

The main reason is vaccines don't work as long as they had hoped. Natural immunity seems to protect forever—for your entire life—long enough that it's really difficult to even test. For vaccines, current estimates range anywhere from 5 to 10 years. It's different for everyone. A natural measles infection used to mean you would never transmit the disease. Now, because only children are getting vaccinated for measles—and the vaccine doesn't protect for more than 10 years—that leaves a significant part of population vulnerable to measles. If only kids get vaccinated, that means everyone else over fifteen years old (and who didn't catch measles as a child) is likely susceptible to measles. That's 80 or 90% of the population that is *unprotected*.

One of the other big problems with vaccines and herd immunity is the way in which certain vaccines mask symptoms of the disease. If you get whooping cough, the buildup of fluid in your lungs will cause you to hack violently in an attempt to get it out. This is a very handy way of mother nature letting you know you are sick. The whooping cough vaccine may prevent you from coughing as much, but it doesn't do much to prevent you from spreading the bacteria. You are still just as infected—and capable of infecting other people—whether you had the vaccine or not.

If you didn't get the vaccine and caught whooping cough, mother nature will give you an obvious warning—violent coughing—a sign that you need to stay away from other people. If you had the vaccine recently, you may be infected, but would have no idea you were carrying a dangerous bacteria. This is why anti-vaxxers believe having friends and family members vaccinated for whooping cough before handling their babies is *very* dangerous. We *want* you to know that you're sick. We *want* you to be able to listen to mother nature's warning cues that you shouldn't be handling a baby.

Every vaccine is different, but there are others that cause similar problems and mask the symptoms of the disease so that you might not realize you're infected. The 95% herd immunity threshold is a meaningless number that has been raised many times with no change in measles outbreaks. China raised the number to 100% in their country for many years and continued to see cases of measles. And remember, that number was originally claimed as capable of eradicating the disease—not controlling outbreaks. If the vaccine protected indefinitely, or every single person got a vaccine every 5 years, it might start to make a difference. For a trivial disease like measles, a once in a lifetime natural infection (with essentially zero risk) sounds like a much better option to the anti-vaxxer.

In summary, when it comes to herd immunity, it hasn't ended up working the way doctors thought it would. Many vaccines don't work for long enough to make a true difference, and many vaccines don't protect against the spread of disease, anyway. If all vaccines could prevent the spread of disease, and they worked for more than a few years, perhaps herd immunity might actually work.

As it stands, every vaccine and every disease are different. Some don't work at all, others work in a very limited way, and still others actually work *against* the herd immunity concept. This is a lot to take in, but it's important that you understand the truth about herd immunity. It's used as an excuse for so many unnecessary vaccines by people who mean well but are horribly misinformed.

I'm guessing you may have one more question—one more thing that's bothering you about all the information I've given you about vaccines. If all of this is true, then why do doctors not know, right? Why do they continue to administer them to so many children—even their own children—if they are really this dangerous or unnecessary?

The answer to this question—the last thing I'm going to talk about—will definitely surprise you.

But doctors!

"But my doctor said vaccines were safe!"

"My doctor said all of her children got their vaccines and nothing happened to them!"

This is probably the most common refrain of anyone who has just begun to question vaccines. Doctors—the ultimate authority on vaccines, right? Who could know more about vaccines than doctors, the ones who administer them every day? I did some research into this and was shocked at what I discovered.

The fact that nothing happened to their children is not surprising. Problems from vaccines don't happen to everyone, and even when something does happen, it might be weeks, even months later. Either way, vaccines are almost never blamed, even when there's an obvious connection. I have seen parents proudly display their children as the recipients of having safely undergone vaccination with no problems, despite their obvious eczema and ongoing gut issues—two known side effects of vaccines.

Doctors say vaccines are safe because they are *taught* they are safe. Until something happens to a doctor's own children—when they see their child change overnight after a vaccine—they will insist that vaccines are nearly incapable of causing harm. The horrible irony is that many of the illnesses they attempt to treat every day can be traced back to reactions to a vaccine, a topic I cover in-depth in another book of mine called *Crooked:Man-made Disease Explained*—a book about how the crooked smiles and misaligned eyes people often see their children develop after vaccines are just the tip of the iceberg of vaccine damage.

If your child starts on an antibiotic and later that day develops hives or nausea, you can guarantee the doctor is likely to take your child off that antibiotic and try something else. If your child receives multiple vaccines and begins having seizures that next day, your doctor is likely to tell you it has nothing to do with the shots and is just a coincidence. If you press them hard and ask them to figure out why your child is suddenly having seizures, they are likely to tell you, "Sometimes we just don't know why these things happen."

Doctors are reluctant to admit vaccines cause problems because a couple of reasons. For one, they have no other tools at their disposal to try and prevent disease. If your child has problems with a particular antibiotic, there are almost always many others they can try—same for most medicines. However, if your child appears to react poorly to a vaccine, the doctor is out of options for protective care (not a problem for anti-vaxxers of course, but that is another story). Another reason they don't like pointing at vaccines as the source of a problem—their side effects can last forever. When you stop taking medicines, both the effects *and* side effects generally stop. Because a vaccine's effects are supposed to last for many, many years, the side effects also can.

If something bad happens to your child after vaccines, doctors have very few options to deal with it. Doctors know this and are obviously going to point towards something other than what they did as the cause for this traumatic event. It's human nature—I'd probably do the same thing.

Finally, the really strange thing about doctors (and

nurses) and vaccines—they are not taught much about them in school. Hardly anything, actually. Compared to the hundreds of hours an anti-vaxxer is likely to have spent studying vaccines, most health care providers know next to nothing. They learn a lot about disease and the immune system and assume that vaccines interact similarly. Unfortunately, they don't. As I mentioned about the ACT problem with the whooping cough vaccine, they are very different. Physicians may spend a few hours learning the schedules recommended by the government, and spend a few hours learning which vaccines should be administered subcutaneously (under the skin) as opposed to intra-muscularly. Beyond that, they learn almost nothing about vaccines.

I was so confused by hearing this, I bought every book listed on the medical curriculum of a prestigious medical school. I even bought some auxiliary books that were not required but on the optional, "recommended" reading list. After going through each and every book on the list—over thousands and thousands of pages—there were only 4 pages that talked about how vaccines work! There were 11 pages that listed the vaccine schedule recommended by the government, but besides that, *4 pages* that talked about vaccines.

I made a video about it, showing the books and how little a prestigious medical school's curriculum spent teaching about vaccines. Many doctors and nurses got in touch with me to confirm this had been their experience in medical school. Of course students learn more than what is taught from their schoolbooks, but I imagine the disparity continues into their classroom and residencies.

Once I understood that doctors and nurses learn very little about vaccines in school, I began to realize why they are so hostile to people like myself who ask honest questions about them. I have written books on the subject, but there are many, many amateur anti-vaxxer mothers and fathers out there who are much, much smarter than me. Any of us could easily stump an average pediatric doctor or nurse on vaccines with some of our common knowledge.

This is not to brag in any way on our intellects, because doctors are some of the smartest people I know—it is simply to indicate how little they actually know about vaccines in particular. If we were to have a contest on anatomy, disease, or which drug to use for a certain problems? Physicians would absolutely beat me all day and night long. When it comes to vaccines, unfortunately even a moderately informed anti-vaxxer is likely to know much more than they do.

I understand that this is going to be very hard for you to accept. Doctors are held high up on a pedestal and we place so much faith in them as they take care of our children. It is a sad state of affairs that the thing they inject into nearly every child that comes into their office, many, many times, whether they are sick or not—they know almost nothing about. This ignorance is usually visible when you question them about the particulars of a vaccine—or vaccine reaction—surfacing as anger or belittlement.

They may tell you a horror story of a child that had tetanus or pneumonia—something they may have seen years ago in their residency at an ER—as anecdotal evidence of the horrors of vaccine preventable disease. This is a blatant attempt to scare you into vaccinating, and it often works. Many parents are unprepared for the amount of bullying they are likely to encounter when even trying to delay a single vaccine. It is a horrible relationship doctors have established with their pediatric parents when honest questions about vaccines are so routinely attacked and met with anger. If your doctor or nurse responds in this way, clearly they don't have your child's best interests in mind. I would snatch your child from the room and not look back. They're working for you, not the other way around, and won't have to deal with the ill effects of a vaccine gone wrong. In fact, they would profit from it.

If you're still reading along, I can guarantee that your head is spinning by now—so much new information that conflicts with what you've been told your whole life. It is a lot to take in, and I've barely touched the surface of the actual situation. Read on just a bit more, and I'll give you some idea as to where to go from here—there are growing numbers of parents who are opting out of vaccines for their children and you are not alone!

Closing thoughts

It can feel frightening to contemplate skipping vaccines for your children. We have been told our whole lives that they are the only thing standing in between certain death and a lifetime of happiness. Unfortunately, the reality is much, much different. Vaccines are a barbaric practice that I am convinced will be a medical relic of the past within a few decades. Imagine restraining your children on a table and purposefully injecting them with modified disease. Take away the linoleum floor, the fluorescent lights and blue scrubs. In any other setting, this practice might feel like a Satanic ritual. For some reason, we have grown to accept this as a natural and acceptable process to put our children through.

In the United States, children are made to go through this procedure dozens of times—often times kicking and screaming the whole way, requiring multiple nurses to pin them down. All in hopes the vaccine *might* protect them from a disease they *might* get that most of humanity never feared before the vaccines. It's truly insanity—from an anti-vaxxer's perspective, at least.

Knowing that most diseases ceased to be dangerous long before vaccines arrived on the scene, knowing that the appearance and disappearance of polio coincided perfectly with extremely dangerous pesticides that were often sprayed directly onto children, and knowing that vaccines are so poorly safety-tested and contain ingredients I'd never let my children ingest (let alone be injected into them), not vaccinating is a very easy decision.

I am not ignorant to the danger of certain infections. I have studied them and respect the harm they can sometimes cause. I also have faith that modern medicine could take care of things if something bad happened. I am suspicious that the ingredients in vaccines are responsible for many of the new neurological and auto-immune conditions that have appeared over the last 100 years.

As a result, I am an anti-vaxxer. You may go on to skip the polio vaccine, or one or two of the others, or you may go on to follow the Dutch or Swedish vaccine schedule, but whatever your choice, the research you do now will no doubt improve the future health of your children. Unfortunately, you cannot trust the information that comes from most health care providers or government health officials. They do not mean any harm to your children, but if history is any guide, they will be the very last to admit the vaccines are causing problems.

This very minute, these two groups are recommending pregnant women get the flu and TDaP shots, even though they have not been safety-tested in pregnant women. The TDaP shot they recommend contains a large amount of aluminum, something you would never willingly allow into your developing fetus for any other reason. This one recommendation, which your doctor will also strongly suggest despite there having been no safety-tests performed, should be a strong indicator of the recklessness in which health care providers treat vaccines.

The Hepatitis B vaccine they will try to inject in your newborn—for a disease they are unlikely to get (unless you test positive for it)—contains a large amount of aluminum. Other countries do not recommend this vaccine. I would consider looking into skipping this vaccine. It is a needless risk for such a young infant.

Finally, I feel that I have to warn you about a few things. You may have already sensed this, but if you do begin to question vaccines, you should be ready to be treated very differently. Most physicians know little about vaccines, yet hold them in a revered place above all other medicines. If you question any of their knowledge on vaccines, or give any indication you may be suspicious about their safety, be prepared to be treated poorly.

I wish that I could say doctors and nurses responded positively to these questions and concerns, but they often react very unprofessionally. Most pediatricians receive generous kickbacks from insurance companies—so long as all of their patients are fully vaccinated. If the percent of their fully vaccinated patients drops below a certain number, they can lose their *entire* compensation. As a result, doctors (and their nurses) are *very* aggressive about vaccinating every child that walks through the door, even if they are clearly sick and should be nowhere near a vaccine.

Many pediatric practices will "fire" you if you do not follow their vaccination program perfectly. They will claim they are doing this out of a concern for the safety of the other patients at the clinic. This is not true. Most are simply trying to protect the generous kickbacks they get from insurance companies. If you are going to cause "problems" by skipping or delaying certain vaccines, you might cost them hundreds of thousands of dollars.

Because of this, many parents go to a family doctor or pediatric chiropractor for check-ups. These physicians don't normally have the kickback programs hanging over their heads and aren't as aggressive about forcing needless vaccines on your family. If you don't already know this, the pediatric "well visits" that doctors request your baby for are really just shot visits. Nurses will weigh them, move their arms around, and check some other development milestones, but it's nothing you couldn't do yourself at home.

New parents are nervous and feel like they have to see a doctor every few weeks just to make sure everything is okay, but the reality is these visits are to facilitate more vaccines and little else. They will really push these visits hard. If you interview a pediatric doctor, tell them you're not interested in the first year of well-child visits just to see their reaction. Tell them you'll come to them if your child is sick (a novel concept, I realize) and nothing else. You may be surprised at their reaction.

If it is legal for you to do so, I would use the audio recorder function on your phone and record your interactions with your doctor or nurse. It may be helpful after you meet with them to review what they told you, especially if anything they said was in a threatening tone.

This is an unfortunate reality of having children within the context of a modern medical system. If you don't play along completely with the vaccine game, you will be a square peg in a round hole and will have to learn to be very aggressive in the way you present yourself. I hate things are this way. I remember when doctors and nurses were happy to listen to your concerns and respect your maternal instincts about what medical procedures were appropriate for your children.

As I mentioned earlier, I have just scratched the surface on the truth about vaccines. There are many other things that I haven't spoken about that will probably shock you. In the final section, I'm going to list a couple of people and places that will help you make informed decisions about how to handle vaccinations with you and your family. I wish the best for you and your family and truly hope you are able to have happy, healthy lives free of neurological, chronic and autoimmune disease.

Resources

There are a lot of excellent, scientific, well-researched resources available to educate yourself more thoroughly on vaccines. Here are just a few to help you get started.

Books
Dissolving Illusions, Suzanne Humphries and Roman Bystrianyk
Vaccines: A Reappraisal, Richard Moskowitz MD
What About Immunizations? Cynthia Cournoyer
Crooked:Man-made Disease Explained, Forrest Maready
The Moth in the Iron Lung, Forrest Maready

Websites
National Vaccine Information Center: www.nvic.org
JB Handley Blog: jbhandleyblog.com/home/onlyvaccineguide
Vaxtruth: vaxtruth.org
Informed Consent Action Network: www.icandecide.org

Facebook
Vaccine Education Network: facebook.com/vaccineeducationnetwork

Additional copies of this book may be available for bulk purchase at: myincredibleopinion.com. Check Amazon if they are not listed on that site.

About the Author

Forrest Maready is a historian, researcher, and author who, along with his wife, has spent the last few years of his life focusing on the underlying causes of the neurological, autoimmune, and chronic illnesses of the modern age. His book, *Crooked:Man-made Disease Explained* chronicles the medicinal metals— mercury and arsenic—of the 1800s, and how they became even more insidious as aluminum and mercury began to be injected directly into the body at the turn of the century.

The Moth in the Iron Lung tells how an invasive species escaped from Boston, Massachusetts, and a new pesticide invented to stop its spread led to the deadly outbreaks of polio across the Northeastern United States at that time.

He currently maintains a popular Facebook and YouTube series called "My Incredible Opinion"— short, educational, and often humorous videos that attempt to explain the truth about vaccines and disease.

Maready spent much of his professional career working in the film and television industries as an editor, sound engineer, animator, and composer. He attended Wake Forest University, studied religion and music, and lives with his wife and son, along with their dog and cat along the beaches of coastal North Carolina.

Notes

Unvaccinated

Made in the USA
Las Vegas, NV
02 November 2024

11004032R00059